READ *Your* BODY

Claire Connellan

authorHOUSE®

AuthorHouse™ UK
1663 Liberty Drive
Bloomington, IN 47403 USA
www.authorhouse.co.uk
Phone: UK TFN: 0800 0148641 (Toll Free inside the UK)
       UK Local: 02036 956322 (+44 20 3695 6322 from outside the UK)

Published by AuthorHouse 09/23/2020

ISBN: 978-1-7283-5374-6 (sc)
ISBN: 978-1-7283-5375-3 (hc)
ISBN: 978-1-7283-5373-9 (e)

Author's Note

What brings me to this chapter. I never thought I would write a book, become an author. Life is a journey and we take many roads with twists and turns, bumps and straight roads. I hope my book will help one deal and cope with areas in their life that can become painful and difficult. I was blessed with the gift of friendship when areas of my life became almost too hard to bear. Family and friends that one can speak comfortably with and can trust are essential. Sometimes we do not realise that this is possible because we get so angry and fed up. We cause a blockage and fail to express our emotions. I believe we have many good friends who support us in different ways throughout our journey, showing care, love and an abundance of kindness and joy. I would like to thank all these fabulous people that have come into my life, all from different paths and helped me to grow stronger and become the person I am today. We can choose to listen and learn from many people in life that will give us the knowledge to be that amazing person, growing, nurturing and creating inner peace, contentment and beauty within. This book is covered from the start to the end with tips and techniques that I have studied and implemented into my life and in all aspects of my daily living with my family, career and my choice of living. I refer to these rituals and methods.

I would like to refer to this book as a source of guidance, a little reminder to stay on this journey of healing and goodness. This is a book that we can look at when things are difficult, dark and painful, it will help the reader to find the strength to persevere. Thank you to all those wonderful people who have helped me get here today.

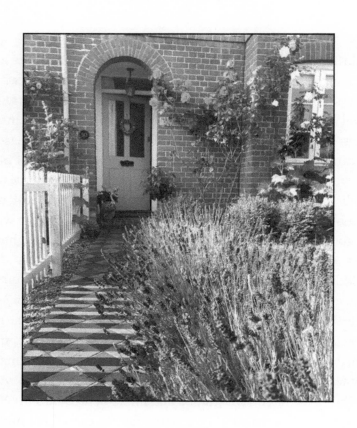

Mission Statement

Look good in the inside, look better on the outside.

Over 95% of the world's population have health concerns.

I am Claire, a health practitioner for 25 years and a tutor in the Department of Health, Beauty and Well-Being.

I am on a mission to share simple ideas, routines, knowledge and beliefs that I have seen and felt myself in my own practice and personally throughout the years, giving an insight on how the body works to create awareness of the connection between the mind, body and spirit of a human being.

I am eager and delighted to share these ideas, techniques, stories to help enhance and encourage mental and physical health, sharing personal methods that one will use daily, weekly or monthly to keep balanced and strong for every event in one's journey through life. During our time on earth we can learn from our mistakes and grow stronger and happier or we can allow life to erode our beautiful personalities and bring us into a miserable space. How our body internally feels and gives visual signs on the external being, what happens when we over think again and again, causing negative thoughts and creating a feeling of misery, thinking far too much about something or someone. How can we put this out of our minds, become positive and happy?

I was inspired to write this book to help others to have a clear vision and feeling of comfort both physically and mentally and to appreciate and understand our feelings at all times. This is a guide to improve one's well-being that is in a state of weakness at the moment and finding it difficult to move forward, or that offers wholesome advice encouraging vitality, harmony and prosperity for a person that is on medication, feeling pain in areas of the body and frightened of serious ill-health. It also offers advice to a person that lies awake at night feeling sadness in his/her heart and failing to have a focus or drive for life. It offers advice to a person that gets overwhelmed, anxious and cannot explain and understand what is happening. It also aims to offer advice to a person that gives away his/her power and strength to be popular amongst his/her peers and offers advice to a person that serves everyone else before serving themselves. Finally this is a guide that offers advice to a person that never listens to or sees one's body and mind in the way that one should and also gives advice to a person that might be attracting the energy of negativity into a life that is causing pain and suffering.

I believe life is precious and a gift. We experience challenging times at different stages and that can be a worry, causing ill-health and strain from family and financial difficulties but one can get support and strength from within by keeping focused and care for oneself taking a guided walk throughout this book and learning how to love, understand and appreciate the most important person which is you.

Make that space today to self-care, self-nourish and build that beautiful soul. One deserves to become comfortable, peaceful, calm and strong by believing in oneself and tuning into the mind and body.

In the past I have overloaded myself with projects trying so hard to get the correct balance. This caused my body and mind to become out of harmony with myself. I changed my life completely for the better. I'm now living a much more harmonious lifestyle that is full of goodness and fulfilment by daily incorporating meditation, yoga, pilates, healthy food, family, friends along with a career I love and treasure. At first it seemed impossible to balance myself appropriately, but I found it successful by taking baby steps and getting support. You can get there too.

"Love yourself by giving your body and mind respect, nourishment, healing and replenishment"

Wishing you an abundance of growth and happiness in all aspects of your life.

Contents

Chapter 1

The Mind and Body Connection

The body and mind are intimately intertwined both physically and emotionally. This is known as mind – body connection. One's brain and organs are constantly communicating with each other. Our minds when out of balance will cause pain in the body. This means our beliefs, feelings, thoughts and experiences can positively and negatively affect our biological functioning. Our minds will affect how healthy or unhealthy the body feels. We can feel tightness, soreness, weakness in the body due to the mind and body being unbalanced.

My eleven-year-old son once said to me that to judge a game of hurling he will visualise where the sliotar {hurling ball} needs to be placed and it is his mind that will make it happen. "Wow". There is a young man realising that the mind controls the physical happenings of **his** body and I thought to myself it is a gift to naturally understand the mind and body signal.

Out of Balance will cause pain.

While the conscious mind is silent, the subconscious mind never rests or sleeps. Many answers come to us as we sleep. One becomes what one thinks and feels.

Mary wanted to purchase a certain style house; she was longing to live in this beautiful old- style cottage but unfortunately the price was not affordable for Mary. She grew very sad, angry, humiliated and anxious believing that she would never get this ideal home. She started to suffer from severe stomach pain. Mary had never paid attention to her emotions. She had no idea what to do and where to go for help. This was a sign that Mary was lacking confidence in her ability and had negative thoughts about her future. Due to feeling miserable and worried, her stomach muscles became tight from over thinking and disgust, leading to excess inflammation internally and causing discomfort and pain.

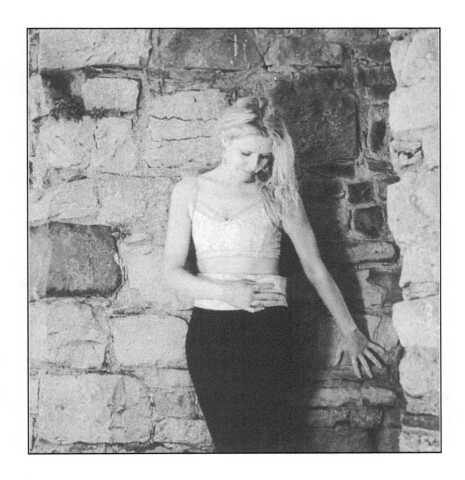

Affirmation

"EXPAND YOUR MIND, STRENGTHEN YOUR INNER BEING, YOUR SOUL AND SPIRIT"

Recognise the signs that the Mind and Body is unbalanced.

False hunger:

Feeling hungry too often reaching for convenient foods when it becomes a habit and eating food that is fattening, it will make one feel heavy and sluggish giving a feeling of laziness and lack of vitality.

Emotional outbursts: Not thinking of what and how one is expressing oneself, lashing out and spreading toxic vibes that communicate in a negative and hurtful way.

Biting your lip: Picking and biting the lip is a sign of frustration, causing an out of control feeling.

Palpitations: This is a rapid increase of one's pulse, a long period of palpitations will affect the normal heart rate and if neglected will lead to heart disease. Palpitations can arise when one becomes anxious and stressed out. One could be aware of the reason or possibly not, begin to monitor the pattern and this will give one a deeper insight. Be patient.

Biting nails: This is a sign of over-thinking and stressing over someone or something in one's life, becoming frightened and nervous of a present situation, lacking patience and self-love.

Memory loss: This can be a foggy mind. Everything becomes unclear, one's system has become overwhelmed and the mind is racing day and night allowing no relaxation. One loses clarity, focus and becomes lost in the pace of life.

Low and High blood pressure: Both can be extremely dangerous to one's health and if one doesn't seek medical help it can lead to heart disease or a stroke, one can experience a feeling of extreme heat and body coldness, a dizzy feeling in the head with confusion and restfulness.

Poor sleeping habit: There are many reasons that can contribute to poor sleeping. **It can be habit-forming. It trains** one's mind to stay active late at night. It gives no space to slow down away from mobiles, laptops, work. Eating late at night will not allow inner workings to slow down and lying down when one feels full will lead to poor digestion, excess acid and a full mind.

Extreme high energy: Imagine a car when it is driven at a high speed every day, what happens? It becomes worn out looking, ages quickly and dated. The human being needs care and nourishment, if one has extreme high energy, it is out of balance. There are many reasons why one keeps moving.

This can lead to burn out and a hormonal imbalance which takes many years to rebuild.

High and low mood: The foods, type and colour, the taste can have an effect on our mood, one can have a high mood when eating fresh healthy foods, one can have a low mood when eating heavy greasy foods. The pleasure of company is important to a high or low mood. When one is surrounded with good vibes and positive energy contentment follows. When in company of negativity and boredom with lack of vitality, one's mood is lowered. Surround yourself with healthy foods and good company.

Weak limbs: Have you heard the sign "I'm weak at the limbs", this can be a sign of being overwhelmed with joy or a sign that the body is losing inner strength with nervous energy and fear.

Sugar cravings: A balanced diet creating efficient goodness for the mind and body will keep away the sugar cravings preventing the energy slumps. It can be provided by eating well and daily exercise.

Headaches/ Migraines: Can become a common occurrence in one's life when the mind and body is out of balance. It is caused by dehydration, a lack of minerals and vital vitamins.

Skin flare up: Can lead to lack of self-confidence and sadness. It can destroy natural beauty and cause one to become withdrawn and insecure. Flare ups can be linked to malnutrition, stress, poor sleep and extreme temperatures.

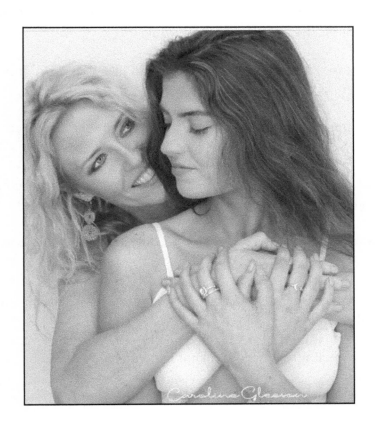

What is Skin Hunger?

Skin Hunger means being touch starved. It is when a human being experiences little or no touch from other humans. This can have a major negative impact in one's life. The power of touch helps to release hormones, serotonin and oxytocin, reducing levels of stress hormones such as cortisol and adrenalin. Our brain's cognitive and emotional centre helps us to experience many health benefits; however being starved of touch can lead to the following:

Loneliness- experiencing a feeling of sadness, despair, loss and confusion.

Depression- feeling there is nothing to look forward to and one can become very judgemental.

Anorexia – feeling a lack of self-nourishment and self-love beginning to hurt emotionally.

Bulimia- feeling physically ugly and developing an urge towards internal sickness.

Aggressive behaviour – feeling fearful and confused lashing out and not realising why one is so angry.

Anxiety - feeling frightened and not knowing what to do.

Here are some vital tips to make a situation work for you.

Create a daily self-care regime to release happy hormones (positive hormones) such as endorphins, dopamine and serotonin that circulate around the body.

Here are the following guidelines to help deal with skin hunger

I WILL TAKE ACTION

- I will breathe in and out 10 times and count 4 inhalations and 4 exhalations.
- I can go for a mindful walk, run, cycle or swim.
- I can look around and be grateful to be alive.
- I will be happy and smile more, inviting goodness into my life.
- I will love my company and expand my hobbies to keep in touch with my inner-being.
- I will implement healthy good habits that will help to become a strong happy human being.

The power of good habits

These are vital to a healthy mind and body to maximise our physical and emotional well-being.

"Our health is our wealth"

Start practicing good habits such as the following:

- Follow a well-balanced diet full of vitamins, minerals and beautiful bright colours and create an array of simple wholesome foods for nourishment.
- Regular exercise; enjoy this time enhancing and maintaining physical fitness and overall health and well-being.
- Create a daily ritual skin and body care regime to fortify a healthy glow.
- Improve concentration with meditation/mindfulness as often as needed, daily, weekly or monthly. Make some quiet time to rejuvenate and replenish the mind and body.
- Music theory; play an instrument or join a musical group, meeting like-minded people that love the art of music.
- Catch up with friends and family: plan some time to go for a sociable drink or meal with good company.

- Have fun, laugh and stay positive making plans and objectives that accomplish.
- Book a massage to help relax and revitalise the aching muscles.
- Make a date for a trip away, something to look forward to and plan some time out from normal and daily routine.

Affirmation "FIND HAPPINESS TO BE THE HARVEST OF A QUIET PEACEFUL MIND".

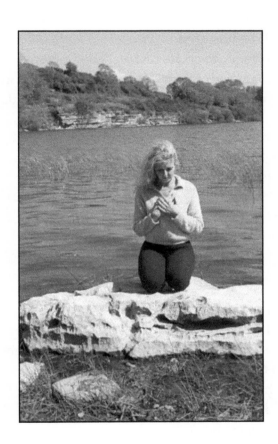

Self- Care - Check in List

Morning Practice

- Gratitude: be grateful to be alive today.
- Visualisation: to earn the aims and objectives planned for the day.
- Get the day off to a good beginning and eat a healthy, nourishing breakfast.
- Self -Hygiene: to create that feel-good factor.
- Dress well: with colours that attract the senses and allow one to feel confident and complete throughout the day.

Daily Practice

- Be mindful of duties..
- Eat healthy food.
- Work out for 30 minutes.
- Drink water between 5 to 8 glasses.

Nightly

- Comfy pyjamas creating 'me time'.
- Go to bed early.
- Visualise something to achieve for a restful night's sleep.
- Mood Lifters such as, read, sing or play music.
- Stretching such as yoga or pilates.
- Meditating to relax the mind and body.
- Breathing in and out.
- Listening to relaxing music.

Check out one's emotional and physical hygiene

If one falls and gets cut the normal thing is disinfect and treat the wound immediately. One will feel better in time.

For emotional and physical hygiene, we will do the same by following these guidelines:

- Seek help immediately when feeling sad and hurt over something from a professional person that can be trusted and respected.
- Create a self-care routine, daily bath or shower, personal hygiene, healthy diet and exercise. Time and nourishment are necessary to give oneself space to heal.
- Deal with the reason one is feeling unwell and move on building resilience and improving quality of life.
- Learn from the experience, forgive and protect oneself from pain in the future, growing stronger and wiser.
- Leave aside issues that will bring one backwards, move forwards with life in a positive and healthy way, onwards and upwards.

Practice the affirmations daily

"I am celebrating life, welcoming peace and moving gracefully along".

"I am safe, I am at peace, I am fulfilled, I am grounded".

Body Talk

"One becomes what one thinks and feels, one looks and acts as one thinks and feels".

Feelings are written all over one's demeanour, expressions are louder than words, the body invites true emotional response, sending signals to how we are truly feeling. One's body participates in a way of either showing or hiding emotions.; crossing one's legs when sitting down, staring at the ground, looking around, lack of eye contact, staring at a phone, lack of engagement. Keeping one's arms across the chest are all signs that one is completely closed off from others.

Keeping the body language in check takes work.

Body Talk Check in List

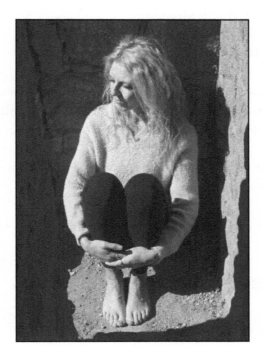

- Daily practice of being mindful regarding one's appearance and attitude.
- Daily exercise: it is vital to do something every day for oneself that one enjoys, for example, incorporating physical activity. This is shown in many ways; a smile, a bounce in the step with enthusiasm and energy.
- Choose clothes to suit one's daily activities. Be confident and comfortable in one's skin and wear a colour that makes natural beauty shine.
  - o **Wear orange and red if feeling the need for protection and safety.**
  - o **Wear blue or purple if feeling the need to stay calm and relaxed.**
  - o **Wear black and brown when feeling the need to be professional and business like.**

- Try to be the best possible person one can be today here and now. Let that internal love, care and kindness come through in actions and words.
- Apply actions to tasks and chores.

Is one under pressure, if so why? What needs to go to create a happy balance, as nothing is forever. Look at life as a book telling a story but it is your biography and each chapter has a different and

unique caption of knowledge and strength that creates a better and balanced person.

If one creates a balanced mind and body this will come through physically.

"Love yourself, nourish yourself, reward yourself".

Chapter 2

Practice Visualisation

Do you see yourself in a positive way, Yes or No?

There are seven micro expressions that one expresses. Although faces are unique, one expresses in a non- verbal way to communicate how one feels.

Anger is expressed in many ways and is associated with the liver which stores blood and detoxifies the body. One's face can appear very discoloured with a high coloured tone when angry. When one is feeling angry it puts the body under pressure increasing blood pressure and causes stagnation of blood flow leading to a feeling of tiredness and exhaustion.

Surprise is expressed when one is shocked, happy or sad. One's eyebrows lift and frown, lines appear on the forehead. It can be a feeling of happiness and delight due to the heart pumping with goodness and lightness or it can be a feeling of pain and tiredness in the chest due to disappointment and upset.

Fear is expressed with sadness and a look of uncertainty, one's colour can appear pale and wizened, legs can become weak and unstable. Kidneys are associated with fear and fright. It is the organ of vitality and energy of life. When out of harmony the body will lack this inner strength.

Contempt shows a lot of internal hurt and pain due to personal experiences, one can develop traits of disrespect and rude behaviour, a continuous pattern of contempt can lead to heart or lung disease.

Sadness is associated with the heart and lungs. It is expressed through crying or dropping away into the background, longing for space to be alone and feeling sorrowful and deeply hurt at the time. When there is a continuous period of sadness in one's life this can cause a low immunity level which leads to frequent colds and flus.

Happiness is expressed with a warm-hearted smile from the soul full of delight and pleasure. One's heart is feeling joyful, face is beaming with enthusiasm and one stands up straight with confidence and pride, full of energy and gratitude for life.

Disgust is expressed with a look of total disapproval of the situation. One stands in a shocked way not understanding what is happening and the reasons why.

An Emotional First Aid Kit

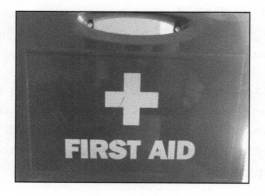

What is an emotional first aid kit?

When I think of a first aid kit I feel confident that it is a box of medical disinfectant lotions and sprays to treat topical cuts, wounds and bandages.

It covers an area to give the abrasion time to heal and while it is healing, the area is clean and safe.

An Emotional first aid kit is related to a physical cut or wound. It is an emotional trauma, so what is needed in the box?

Space

Time is needed away from the situation that has caused this trauma in one's life. This can be done by altering one's mind away from the hurt or physically seeking time away, completely breathing new air and removing oneself from the situation that caused pain.

Nourishment

- Physically and mentally following a good healthy diet full of goodness.
- Exercise to detox the mind and body from the hurt.

Therapy can be received in many ways

1. Book an appointment with a counsellor to speak comfortably about thoughts and feelings, a person one can fully trust.
2. Make the time for a massage, full body, half body, Indian head, foot or hand massage whatever area feels achy and needs nurturing at this time.
3. Book a holiday to seek 'me-time', space and fun immediately, to create happiness and help clear one's mind of negativity and pain.
4. A night out with true friends who will listen and give an uplift; that always works.
5. A book of morning and night-time affirmations to help keep one thinking and feeling positive.

An emotional kit can have an endless list of ways to heal from trauma.

I have practiced this affirmation many times and it works!!

Relax in a quiet and peaceful area, take a deep breathe in and hold for 4 seconds while the abdomen expands.

Relax and exhale letting all the air out, repeat this 10 times. When fully relaxed say this affirmation with hands placed on the heart.

"I believe in myself. I know my self-worth. I am happy and have so much to give. I will care for myself, become true to myself and here and now build a stronger and happier me.

Feel peace and contentment within".

Emotional trauma can have an everlasting damaging effect.

Guilt- taints one's sense of self- belief and stops one from forgiveness.

Anger- affects one's thinking capacity and contributes to serious health conditions.

Sadness- becomes unaware of one's true feelings, thoughts and behaviour

Rejection- lowers self-esteem. One grows ashamed…

Disgust - gives a feeling that one needs to get something internal out of the system. It gives a feeling of nausea.

Fear- develops into a phobia, a feeling of danger and being scared.

Emotions are Contagious.

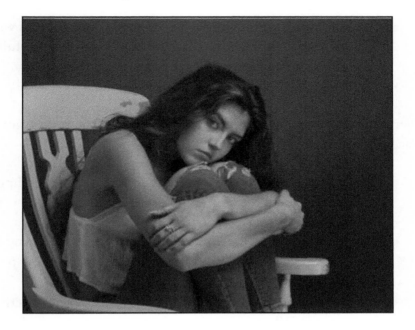

When one meets someone and converses with him/her, one is subconsciously mimicking micro movements of the other person's facial muscles. If one smiles, we smile. If one cries, we feel sad and look sorrowful. If one verbalises one of the seven micro expressions, we can have a positive or negative reaction towards one. This involuntary image matches the other person's sense of feeling. One dwells on it for the entire day.

Some characters can clash with each other and it is unhealthy to be in that company for long periods of time. Circumstances may be difficult. It is important to recognise this feeling and know when it is not safe or just right. Address this awkwardness and move away without judgement.

Here are tips to combat this feeling if it is negative

- Visualise that one is in a gold box of blissful beauty. This will be a protection from any negative vibes and one can gracefully move on with positive energy and day to day routine.
- Understand that it is important to be non-judgemental.

Every human being has a personal story and may not be in a good place at this time.

- Protection is key, choose the company, the surroundings around one and if the vibes from people are negative, there is no need to stay in such an uneasy situation.
- When one is aware and not in a good place, time and space is essential. Take one day at a time to understand the situation and implement self-care into the daily regime.
- Fill the daily schedule with fun and happiness to keep positive and focused. When one notices a decline in energy or feelings, be kind to one self.
- Practice deep breathing as often as possible to release the happy hormone endorphins which liberate natural calming effects in the entire body.

Reading the Face

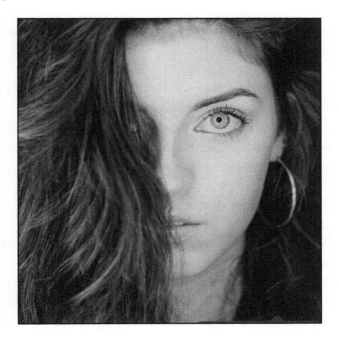

Checking into the reasons why our skin can be aging quickly and becoming sensitive and irritated.

- **Forehead, cheeks and nose** will show signs of worry when one is stressed. This causes a build-up of acid in the digestive tract which leads to inflammation. When stressed one will reach for the unhealthy food which will put the digestive tract under pressure due to causing inflammation internally. When the internal organs become inflamed, this manifests itself in the cheeks, nose and forehead with dryness, sensitivity and discolouration, causing one to touch and rub the skin even more than normal.
- **Eyebrow area** can show signs of gallbladder issues, poor water intake leading to dehydration. If one is consuming a poor diet, the area around the brows can become sensitive, dry and sore to touch, looking old and flaky.

Cheeks can have blocked pores and blemishes due to dirty pillowcases and over-use of a mobile phone. To avoid blocked pores and spots that become infected, wash the pillow-case weekly and clean the surroundings of the phone.

- **Ears** can get blemishes and become blocked with wax due to a hormonal imbalance and a lot of stress in one's life.
- **Jaw-line and chin area** blocked with comedones (blackheads) and milia (white-heads), normally caused by a hormonal imbalance and a poor diet.

Why encountering a lot of stress leads to skin aging?

When one is stressed, the body requires extra energy to get through the stressful situation. So it releases the hormone cortisol (stress hormone). Cortisol inhibits insulin and releases sugar and fat from storage sites throughout the body into the blood for use as energy. The released sugar molecules are vulnerable to glycation, the more sugar one eats, the more AGE (Advanced Glycation End) one develops. An accumulation of AGE damages adjacent protein collagen and elastin which are the fibres that keeps skin firm and elastic.

What are the signs to recognise when the skin is prematurely aging?

- Dark circles around eyes
- Puffy eyes
- Saggy skin
- Cellulite
- Stretch marks
- Skin tags and lesions
- Broken capillaries
- Superficial lines.

Daily TIPS to improve the quality of the skin and take years from the age of the skin

- Improve one's sleeping pattern by getting at least 8 to 10 hours sleep per night.
- Practice daily meditation to give oneself space and time to heal and grow inner peace.
- Increase consumption of anti-oxidants in the diet such as cherry tomatoes, green leafy vegetables such as spinach and kale. Omega 3, 6 and 9 fish oils can be consumed in fish such as organic salmon, tuna and mackerel.
- Improve intake of water, drink a glass of lukewarm water first thing in the morning before one eats to flush out toxins from the large intestine and drink 5 to 8 glasses daily.
- Fresh fruit is a natural energy booster and gives one natural sugar such as berries, bananas, mango and melon.
- A daily skin care regime to keep the skin looking hydrated and protected from the sunrays and pollution.
- Take daily exercise to boost the lymphatic system to eliminate excess toxins internally. Too much acid in the body leads to a feeling of tiredness even when one gets enough sleep. One will feel exhausted and worn out, the stomach will experience bloating and gas and indigestion will lead to extreme flatulence and discomfort.

How to recognise if the body has an over-load of acid?

- Unhealthy skin - such as dermatitis, psoriasis and eczema.
- Unhealthy hair - split ends and dryness.
- Unhealthy nails - causing them to be brittle and weak.
- Sensitive gums and teeth.
- Low energy.
- Poor sleeping pattern.
- Headaches.
- Eye health.
- Poor metabolism.
- Cramps.
- Infections.
- Poor digestion.

Balance the pH level

The human body must keep its **pH** at a range of 7.35 – 7.45 on a scale of 0 to 14. The body is built to naturally maintain a healthy balance of acidity and alkalinity. Being too acidic affects the entire mind and body.

How to balance the pH in the body

- Avoid the intake of processed foods, artificial sweeteners.
- Avoid sugar in the diet.
- Eat alkaline foods such as greens, fruits, vegetables.

Eat foods as follows: greens, spinach, parsley, kale, watercress, grains and beans, millet and quinoa. Nuts and seeds, almonds, chia powder, sesame seeds, raw fruits, melons, lemons, limes, dates, figs and raisins.

Health Tips for the Mind and Body

"Personal direction is so much more important than speed in one's life, create a clear vision, focus, plan and one can achieve what one desires".

A daily plan keeps one focused. Everything takes work when one begins to make a change to improve and enhance one's well-being. It needs to be tailored to individual needs and demands met comfortably and genuinely. Exercise and healthy food are essential to both one's mind and body but is it enough to keep us balanced, full of nourishment and fulfilment?

"SELF CARE IS THE BEST CARE".

FIND YOURSELF

TRUST

CREATE YOUR SPACE

A hectic life can cause one to lose focus and the meaning of life, learning to cope in a bubble of confusion, despair, panic and fear. Becoming out of balance, pain and trauma manifest in the body in different ways, not listening to the body, not noticing the signs in a physical or mental capacity.

When asked," Do you take care of yourself?" You immediately reply "Yes" without thinking about what it means!

What does it mean to take care of one self?

What does it take?

Self-Care is living a balanced life. Self-care needs to be planned. It is an active choice of living a balanced life both mentally and physically. It refuels our mind and body in areas that work for us, making commitment and putting it into practice. One must learn about oneself and what works for one, how it feels and what to create to achieve that balanced lifestyle.

PRACTICE GRATITUDE

DISCOVER PEACE

BE CALM

Do you feel it is the time to grow and find fulfilment and happiness? Live in the present moment and engage in the never-ending process of self- improvement. Tune into the inner voice, continue to learn, grow and contribute to a life full of gratitude, health and love.

Start focusing on positive inner strength, meditate and create space for self-care and self-love.

YOU ARE WORTH IT.

Find the smile again, is the smile lost? Or is it noticeable? Think about the following!

Do we attract people that are positive? Do we attract good energy and people full of the vitality? **The key is balance and protection**.

I will give clear guidelines that work to keep one from being fearful or bothered about the unknown.

These are some methods to give support in this area:

Create a vision board.

Include

Pictures, memories, affirmations that will start one on the healing journey of clarity and enthusiasm bringing one to colour, creativity, excitement and thoughtfulness.

Write down a daily regime of realistic aims and break it into 3 categories

1. Morning
2. Midday
3. Evening

What is a vision board?

It communicates our concepts and aims to achieve our goals in life and gives us a structure and timeframe to work towards using a collage of images and aims.

VISION BOARD

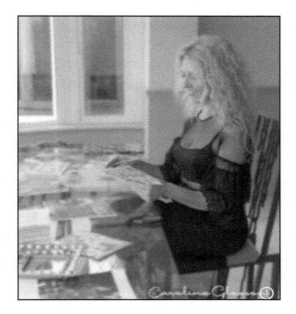

Words of inspiration

- Love
- Peace
- Good Vibes
- Good Life
- Love Friends
- Network
- Fun
- Holiday
- Be creative
- Career
- Exercise
- Positivity
- Dreams
- Image
- Meditate
- Spend quality time with family

Re-Programming one's life here and now.

Life is a journey with many twists and turns.

We can make our journey scenic, creative and playful or we can experience a journey with pain, punishment and despair.

Our body can ache from disappointment. We may not have made time or thought enough about something or someone when we should! Our body can ache and hold on to sadness, fear, grief or worry. We may have held back and didn't make a situation work or didn't make the space for what could have been a priority at that time.

Our body and mind both physically and mentally may be suffering because we are feeling upset and frustrated so we over-eat, over-drink and express emotions in a hurtful way when in pain.

Develop a clear positive vision to get clarity, create magical vibes. When a Vision Board is created for life it will increase motivation, encourage one to aim for success and map out objectives over a duration of days, months and years. A Vision Board provides one with gentle reminders of goals and dreams to aspire to in life-seeking fulfilment to provide growth and happiness.

We all have regrets and questions. Learn from the negatives and make it into something beautiful and positive. Mistakes are part of life. To feel unwell and out of balance at times is normal.

This is the time to learn from the negatives and create a brighter future.

"You are Unique,

You are Powerful,

You are Beautiful".

Chapter 3

Meditate with Me

MEDITATION CREATES SPACE ALLOWING

TIME

CLARITY

LOVE

Meditation will bring a deeper understanding to oneself.

WE ARE ON A JOURNEY; Meditation balances one's left and right brain hemisphere resulting in what is called "Whole Brain Synchronization". The brain is a community of 50 trillion living cells so there are cells in harmony and cells in disharmony which can become manifest in disease. The good news is meditation heals at the molecular level. It creates amazing health benefits in both mental and physical well-being, evolving happiness, focus, creativity, peace, intelligence, will power and contentment. Make space to meditate, learn to practice. Grow deep levels of consciousness.

Meditation unfolds naturally as the mind grows tranquil.

Meditation has no physical movement in the body, the process will happen through guided step by step procedures and tuning into the mind and body without trying to evaluate or rationalise the situation, just go with the flow. There is no correct or incorrect method.

It is a unique practice for one's health. It is a new and fresh experience not a competition.

The following are guidelines to help relax the mind and body:

- Allow one's eyes to close gently.
- When one is ready focus on the feet.
- Feel one's toes relax,
- Let go of tension and tightness.
- Let the mind rest.

Relax the mind, let this feeling spread outwards and downwards, moving into the ankles which will loosen and relax. Relaxation spreads into the calves, knees, getting deeper and deeper, moving into our thighs. Feel the lightness, looseness throughout, carrying on up into the abdomen and chest and neck. Let go of the tension held in the neck. Muscles become looser and looser. Now move into the head, face and eyes, feel a deep relaxation, loosen every little muscle bit by bit, step by step. Feel the tongue relax. Move down the shoulders, feel the tension and tightness leave the body. This wonderful state of relaxation is spreading into the arms, elbows and into every finger, the right thumb and left thumb. The world is moving slowly, it is peaceful and in a state of harmony. Meditation expands the concentration and creates space to tune into our mind and body. Reading the body and being able to visualise our internal organs will allow us to have a deeper understanding of the human body.

AFFIRMATION

"One will not find joy in things or others. One will find it within oneself".

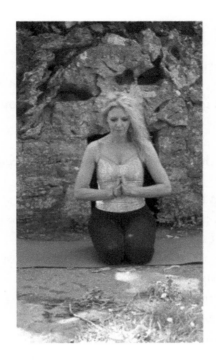

- **SIMPLY BE,**
- **PRACTICE THE POWER OF NOW,**
- **MEDITATION SUITS,**

Below is a

CHECK-IN Questionnaire.

Please answer all questions in relation to how you have felt during the past week.

One can refer to this questionnaire as often as required.

- How often have I meditated?
- When talking to other people, was I aware of their facial and body expressions?
- When I walked outside, was I aware of smells or how the surrounding area looks?
- When someone asked how was I feeling, could I identify my emotions easily?
  o **I should not feel miserable.**
  o **I should not have certain thoughts.**

- Was I aware of what thoughts were passing through my mind?
- If there was something I did not want to think about, did I try many things to get it out of my mind?
- Did I wish I could control my emotions more easily?
- Were there aspects of my behaviour I did not want to think about?
- Did I try many things to clear my negative thoughts? Did I feel the water flow over my skin when I showered?
- Were there memories that I tried not to think about?

Meditation takes practice and respect. Before one starts to meditate choose a comfortable place with soft lighting and surroundings, warm and peaceful, creating space to encourage the mind-set to focus on self-care and growth.

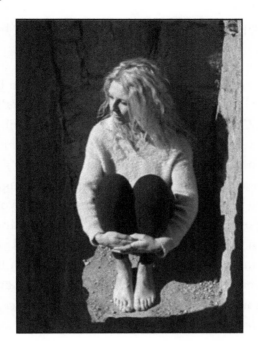

Meditation to help reduce anxiety

https://soundcloud.com/user-702459334/meditation-for-anxiety-

Find a comfortable place away from all distractions. Make this time, make space, gently close your eyes, inhale and exhale taking a deeper breath than you have taken today.

There is nowhere else you need to be, taking a deep breath, inhale, grounding you into the present moment, just here. Well-being is your focus for now. Continue to take slow deep breaths, inhale expanding your lungs. As you inhale feel the journey of the breath. Feel the relaxation go through your body and hold it for a beat, feel the journey of your breath as you continue inhaling and exhaling, notice places you are holding tension. Unfold your brow, unclench your jaw, release tension from your shoulders. Allow your shoulders drop down from your ears, open the left palm and the right hand, feel your legs, relax every muscle in your body. Call to mind a situation that is causing you anxiety even when you feel you are over it. Why are you judging yourself and causing pain? Acknowledge its presence, breathing in and out, let it go, give the story permission to drop away now, notice your mind pushing you harder to hold on to those thoughts and acknowledge that the level of anxiety has decreased. Notice how the anxiety becomes less, a deep breath in and exhale again, a deeper breath, even deeper than the one before, feeling the deep breath, relax, in between the muscles and cells, now even deeper than the one before. Practice this meditation as often as you feel.

Anxiety is when the mind takes over and allows foggy thoughts and frightening feelings. Meditation will focus your mind encouraging inner strength and belief.

Create one's natural ability to heal.

The greatest addiction of all is **'cannot stop thinking'**.

Cannot stop drinking

Cannot stop eating

Meditation is creating space with quiet inner thought.

Over thinking loses the ability to know oneself and to self-care.

Practiced meditation will slow down the over-active mind, create simplicity and calmness.

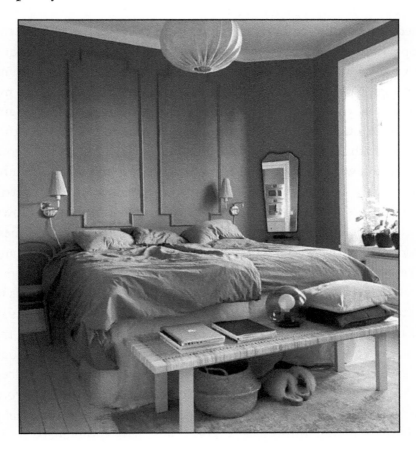

Meditation

Sleep <u>https://soundcloud.com/user-702459334/meditation-for-sleep</u>

Create Headspace.

Let go of the overactive thoughts past and future. Tonight release these feelings, focus on the present moment, let go of negativity and stress to create a powerful deep and relaxing night's sleep.

Welcome to my meditation to create headspace and settle into meditation with me here and now. I **<u>am so grateful</u>** to have the opportunity to guide you to inner peace, to create a safe and tranquil environment. Ensure your room is dark with little light coming through. Now that you are fully prepared, close your eyes, allow my voice to be your guide on this journey. Inhale through your nose and exhale through your mouth, sink deep into your bed. Taking another deep breath, begin to count your breath, one count longer than your exhale allowing each exhale to carry away stress and worry. Breathe slowly in a calming nature, feel the cool air entering your nostril, continue to observe your breath, allow it to naturally slow down breath by breath. Feel the weight of your body and notice the heaviness increase, feel the relaxation flow through your body. Remain still and feel your body going deeper and deeper into a relaxed state. Allow your head to feel heavy, allow your face to relax, your facial expressions to soften, move your awareness to your mouth. Feel the sensations in your mouth. Notice your jaw, lips, upper lip, lower lip, teeth, feel the inside of your cheeks and now all your face as a whole. Feel your body relax, getting deeper and deeper. Feel your body draft into a deep restful position. No need to hold yourself. Let go of every part of your body, feeling every part getting heavier and heavier. You will feel a softening in your **tummy,** legs, knees, feet, hands, shoulders, neck, head, forehead and chest.

Practice this meditation to help to encourage your mind and body to have a restful sleep.

Here are some questions that will help you determine how much you need to listen and follow through step by step guidance to enhance your sleeping pattern.

1. Do you get tired at night-time after your daily chores and look forward to retiring to your bedroom?
2. Do you wake early full of energy to take on the day?
3. Do you sleep straight away after getting into bed or does it take you a while before you can sleep?
4. Do you feel worried at night, knowing that it is going to be difficult to get to sleep, stay asleep or do you get any proper sleep?
5. Do you sleep for a few hours and then wake for a few hours, when it is time to get up in the morning you feel like staying in bed?

Sleep is so important to one's health for both the mind and body. While one sleeps the body heals and recuperates. Poor sleep leads to low immunity causing the mental and physical health to weaken.

Self-Healing Meditation

https://soundcloud.com/user-702459334/meditation-for-selfhealing

Welcome to my meditation to create space for self- healing. Find a comfortable place, warm and relaxing for you. Close your eyes, imagining yourself looking outside of yourself and repeat the following:

I will forgive myself

I will heal my body and mind

I am aware of my feelings

I will find balance

I will relax every cell in my body

Feel the sensations of your breath as you take a deep slow inhalation through your nose counting to 4 and exhale through your mouth counting to 4, allow yourself to breathe, feeling the relaxation flow through your body like a river flowing, letting go of your shoulders, jaw, facial expressions, tension around your brow, mouth, cheeks, let go of the weight of gravity as your body softens and your mind begins the journey of healing.

Begin to observe the path of your breath creating a rhythm of pure relaxation, sending energy fuelled breaths into every cell of your body. Every organ welcomes this vitality, opening up and receiving it with gratitude like a blossoming flower. You are your own best healer realising today here and now how talented and capable you are to heal yourself. Bring your awareness back to your breath focus on a light full of goodness and purity shining up through your feet into your legs, knees and hips spreading across your stomach and chest, shoulders, neck and face. Warmth and healing spreads an array of regeneration and rejuvenation throughout the entire body. The body feels heavier and heavier as you let this power of well-being heal within, embracing the power of self- healing.

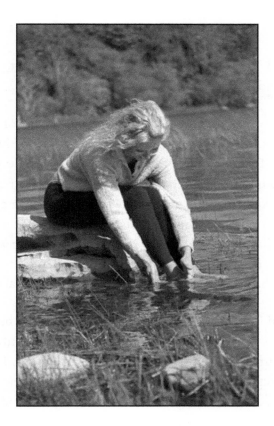

Self-Healing is so important, practice this meditation as often as you need to encourage your mind and body to heal from a trauma or hurt. When one chooses not to address a trauma, this can manifest internally and become a disease. Care for your well-being before it is too late.

Meditation to Release Emotional Pain and Physical Pain

https://soundclouds.com/user702459334/self-healing-to-release-emotional-pain-and-physical-pain

Slowly find a comfortable place, space for you, away from noise, from the outside world. Close your eyes, pay attention to the breath and the rhythm of flow as you inhale and exhale. Inhale pure vitality expanding your lungs and exhale pain, negativity and stress out of your body. Inhale counting to 4 and exhale counting to 4. Imagine a bright ball, it is coloured blue. The ball is at the soles of your feet. Continue to breathe, inhaling and exhaling. This ball is rolling up along your leg and when you feel tightness or discomfort it will stay there, while you inhale and exhale releasing physical pain and emotional pain.

Let it rise and flow away out through your feet, invite healing, create space for your inner wisdom to do work. As this beautiful blue ball rolls over your body, some pain or discomfort arises. Hold it there, inhaling a deep breath and exhaling several times creating space for inner healing. Allow it to surface and flow away. Practice this guided meditation for releasing pain from an emotional or physical happening. This can be used when one is experiencing grief from perhaps a loss of a loved one or multiple losses. One is taken away from one's normal surroundings and left empty and in a place of despair and disbelief. This pain can lodge internally and weaken your immunity leading to ill health. When one practices this meditation it will release the pain, slowly step by step, piece by piece, allowing you to strengthen and heal to live a happier and more contented life.

Move forward with pure inner strength and focus.

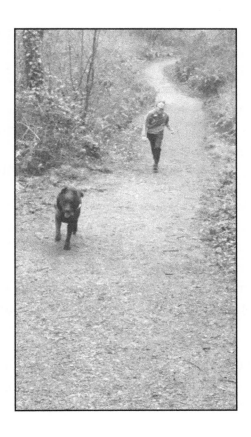

Meditate with Me Starting a healing journey

https://soundcloud.com/user-702459334/meditation-to-start-ahealing-journey

This is priority for you here and now. Whatever you are dealing with whether it is stress or an imbalance that is impeding you from living a full life of contentment. You will begin an inner healing to wipe away this negativity flowing through your cells, erasing and dissolving it bit by bit, starting to facilitate your healing journey of happiness and self- care.

Welcome and I am so grateful to spend this time with you to help you on your journey of healing today. Make yourself as comfortable, safe and at peace as you possibly can, now close your eyes and take a deep breath counting to 4 and exhale counting to 4, repeat by 10.

I invite you to join me on a journey to the wood. This is a beautiful peaceful place full of green grass, trees and blue-bells, continue to breathe as you exhale. I invite you to let go of all the stress lodged in your body step by step. Scan your body, just let go of any tension, tightness, pain in your feet, toes, legs, hips, buttocks, stomach, hands, shoulders, chest and head. Stay here and work through your body, letting any discomfort rise and go.

It is a beautiful day, the sun is shining and you feel this heat on your back and what a wonderful presence of peace is surrounding you. Continue to inhale, relax and exhale any feeling of tiredness and achy feeling throughout your body. Now imagine roots of a tree under your feet, you have connected with water, moss, grass, soil under the ground to create nurturing and nourishment. These are energy roots. You have connected with goodness and will now draw up energy.

This will revitalise your feet, legs, hips, buttocks, stomach, hands, shoulders, chest, neck and head. Breathe out love and contentment feeling grounded and fulfilled to face the world. When I think of healing, I imagine one to be feeling broken and weak. Mind and body barely function and one drags oneself from one day to another. Practice this meditation to start the journey of healing, building and revitalising every cell internally to a healthy and beautiful human being, full of fun, laughter and warmth with a lightness of beauty shining through your actions.

This takes time but it will happen and during this journey of healing. One will realise how strong and capable one is.

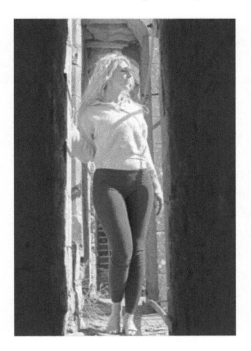

Meditate with Me

Falling in love with yourself

What is self- love?

Meditate with Me

Cutting negativity and welcoming positivity into your life.

We attract people and things to match how we are feeling.

When we are full of negativity, sorrow and thinking of misery, this sends out poor vibes.

This will reflect itself into the universe, it will come to you in abundance.

How can I prevent this from happening to me?

Yes, this takes work, patience and knowledge to have a positive reflection.

Here are some pointers to remember:

1. Lose the tension
2. Walk the Walk
3. Talk the Talk
4. Treat others the way you want to be treated
5. Smell the danger
6. Spot the signs

Affirmation

"**A negative person is hurting, perhaps frightened and has lost control of his/her emotions. It is not you, as you are working at your well-being, like watering a plant to aid growth and beauty, giving it the space to blossom and spread its aroma**".

Chapter 4

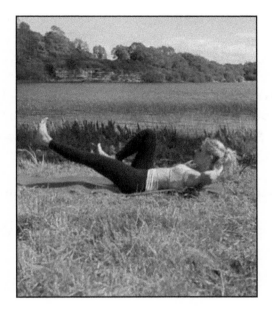

When the body lets down the mind, the mind lets down the body.

The body and mind connection expresses itself in many ways such as holding the weight of the world on your shoulders, feeling dragged down.

'Fed up' signals are signs of the mind moulding the physical being.

We can hold onto negative thoughts and go to bed in a good or bad psychological state. This will be reflected in body tone and tension. It will be reinforced in one's posture and demeanour.

What muscles are responsible for one's posture?

They include muscles in:

- The abdomen
- The lower back
- The buttocks
- The pectorals across the front of the chest
- The trapezius across the back of the shoulders
- The quadriceps thighs
- The calves
- The biceps, the tops of the arms

In this chapter I have a guided step by step routine of stretches to strengthen core muscles. It will improve posture and confidence. Balance the mind and body by improving concentration and facilitating change.

Start your journey today, get fit, strong and more confident.

Spend 30 minutes 3 times a week at home following this simple routine.

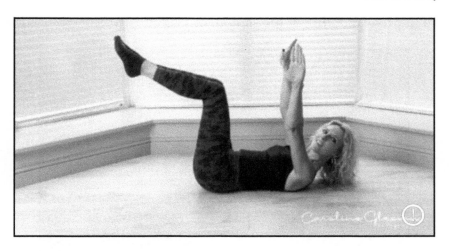

Pilate Techniques and Tips

Gain absolute Balance between Mind and Body = Genuine Normal Health

The aim of Pilates is to focus the mind using controlled progressive and intelligent exercise building strength and flexibility slowly.

The basics of safety when using Pilates:

- Warm up first
- Build up each exercise slowly and systematically
- Take new exercises one step at a time
- If possible, exercise in front of a mirror to check position
- Avoid exercise after eating
- Drink water before and after exercise. If, at any point, breathlessness, a feeling of nausea, back pain or chest pain occurs, stop immediately.

Here are some beginner and intermediate stretches to tone and strengthen your core muscles, transforming the body and improving both mind and body well-being.

To improve mobility of the shoulders

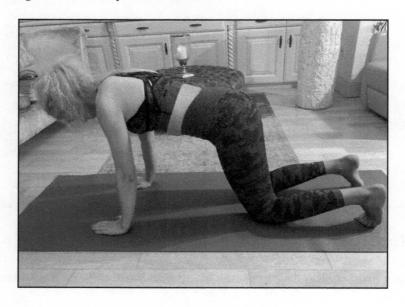

Aim - to strengthen the arms and pectorals

Start on your hands and knees

Keep your arms just over a shoulder's width apart

Raise your back parallel with the floor

Extend your back, long as possible

Breathe in

Tighten your abdominal muscles

Press your chest towards the floor

Breathe out

Push back to the start position

Repeat 10 times

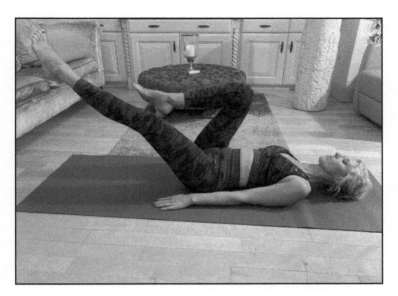

Aim – to develop spinal stability

Repetitions 10 left and 10 right side

Lie on your back

Arms by your sides

Bend your knees

Legs hip distance apart

Contract your abdomen

Drop your shoulder blades to the floor

Relax your chest

Breathe in

Lift your right knee towards your chest until your knee is above your hip

Breathe out

Return to start position, keeping abdominals contracted

Change legs

Repeat 10 times on each leg

Lean Forward Bending

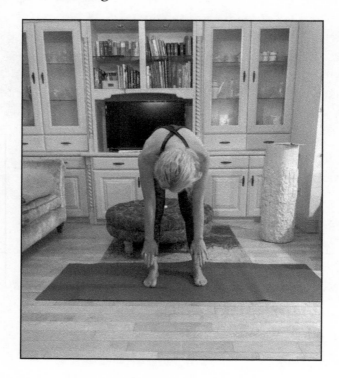

Aim - to develop flexibility in the spine and hips

Repetitions 10

Stand upright in a good posture

Place your feet a hip's width apart

Breathe out

Bend forwards from your hips

Stick your bottom out and maintain a straight spine

Breathe in.

Tighten your buttocks and use your hips to return to the standing position

Repeat 10 times

Leg Extension

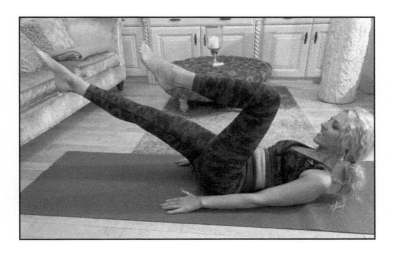

Aim – to develop spinal stability and control of the lumbar vertebrae

Repetition 10 right and 10 left side

Lie on your back,

Arms loosely by your hips

Keep your knee a hip width apart,

Bend your left knee

Contract the abdomen

Drop your shoulder blades to the floor

Relax your chest

Breathe in

Lift your right knee to a 45-degree angle whilst keeping your leg straight

Breathe out

Return to start position,

Keep abdominals contracted

Change legs

Repeat 10 times on each leg

Leg Pull Back

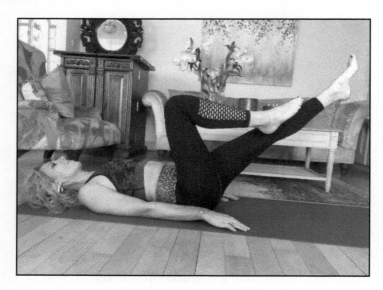

Aim - to develop stability in the shoulders and upper arms, to stretch the hamstrings and increase flexibility in the hips

Repetition 6 right and 6 left leg

Start from a sitting position, legs straight in front and together

Place your hands on the floor, slightly behind your hips

Point your toes gently

Breathe in

Slowly bring your right knee up, sliding your foot lightly along the floor and raising it slightly

Keep your hip square and back straight

Breathe out

Slide your foot back to the starting position

Change leg

Repeat 6 times on each leg

Leg Pull Down

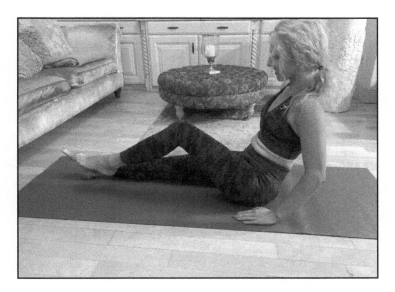

Aim – to develop stability in the shoulders and upper arms to stretch the lower leg muscles

Repetitions 5 right and 5 left leg

Start on your hands and knees

Keep your arms just over a shoulder's width apart

Raise your back parallel with the floor

Extend your back as long as possible

Breathe in

Tighten your abdominal muscles

Breathe out, lifting one leg

Hold the leg straight and parallel to the floor at hip height for a count of five

Return to start position and change legs

Repeat 5 times on each side

Lunge

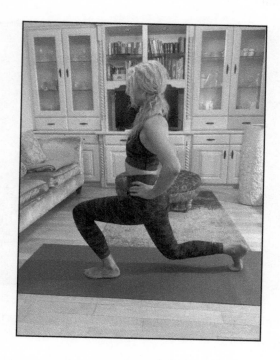

Aim - to tone the buttocks and improve hip mobility

Repetition 5 left and 5 right

Start in a good posture, feet a hip's width apart

Take a comfortable step forward, keeping your body upright

Breathe in

Bend your leg until your thigh is just past parallel to the floor

Breathe out

Push through your front foot to return to upright

Change legs

Repeat 5 times on each leg

Mermaid

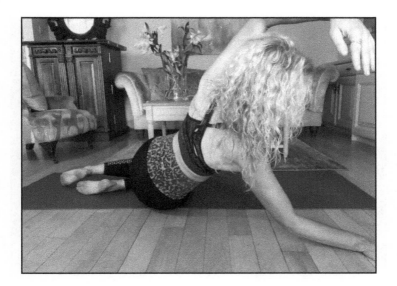

Aim - to strengthen the core musculature

Repetitions 5 left and 5 right side

Kneel on the floor then drop to the right-hand side so that you are sitting on your right hip with your feet behind you

Breathe in

Tighten your abdomen

Reach to the right side, placing your right elbow as close to the floor as you can

At the same time, take your left arm over your head as far as you can

Breathe out

Breathe in

Staying on your right hip, bend to the left, taking both arms as before

Breathe out

Change to sitting on your left hip and work in the opposite direction

Repeat 5 times on each hip

Side Leg Lift

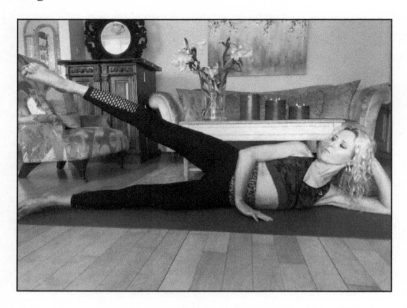

Aim – to tone the legs and strengthen the hips

Repetitions- 5 left and 5 right leg

Lie on your left side with your head propped in your left forearm, maintaining a straight line along the floor, legs together (right above left leg), and toes pointed

Tighten your abdomen

Breathe in, lifting your right leg straight upwards

Bend your foot up, breathe out and bring your leg down slowly, imagining a resistance

Repeat 5 times on each side

Single Leg Circles

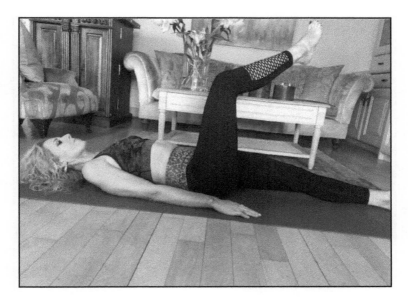

Aim – to improve mobility and strengthen the legs

Repetitions- 5 left leg and 5 right leg

Lie on your back in a good posture, legs straight and together, and arms by your sides, palms down Tighten your abdomen

Raise your right leg vertically so that your knee is directly above your hip

Breathe in and circle your leg anticlockwise

Breathe out and circle your leg clockwise

Repeat 5 times on each leg, alternating sides

Single leg kicks

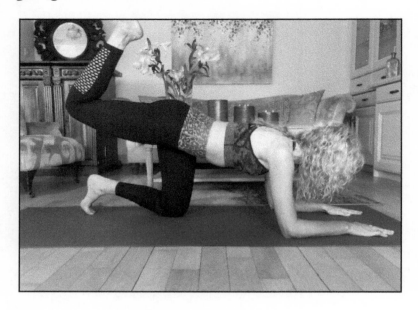

Aim – to strengthen the hamstrings and lengthen the spine and hips

Repetitions 10 left and 10 right

Lie on your front with your elbows under your shoulders to support your body, hands at your sides Tighten your abdomen, buttocks and inner thighs

Breathe in, raising your right foot

Breathe out, pulsing your right heel twice towards your right buttock

Return your leg to the start position

Change legs

Repeat 10 times on each leg

Curl Ups

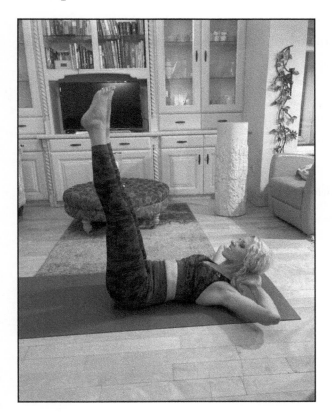

Aim – To strengthen the abdominal muscles

Repetitions 10 times.

Lie on your back

Bend your knees

Keep your feet flat on the floor, 45 cm apart

Keep your arms by your sides, palm down

Breathe in

Lengthen the back of your neck

Contract your abdomen

Put your hands behind your head, elbow flat

Breathe out

Raise your upper body

Leave the bottoms of your shoulder blades on the floor

Extend your legs straight

Breathe in

Extend your spine and neck

Hold the position for a few seconds

Breathe out

Return to start position, leaving your hands behind your head

Repeat 10 times

Double Leg Stretch

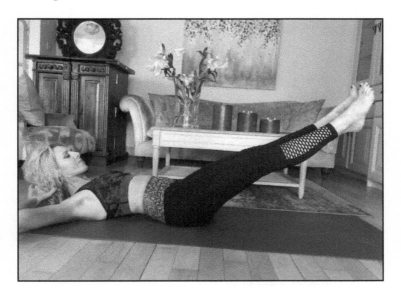

Aim – to develop co-ordination and strengthen the abdominal muscles

Repetitions – 8

Lie on your back

Raise your knees so that they are above your hips

Lift your head from the floor, lengthening the back of your neck

Place your hands just below your knees

Breathe in

Extend your arms wide, over your head

Straighten your legs, lengthening the muscles to a 45-degree angle from the floor

Breathe out

Contract your legs and buttocks and return your knees to the start

Circle your arms back to your knees

Repeat 8 times

The Bridge

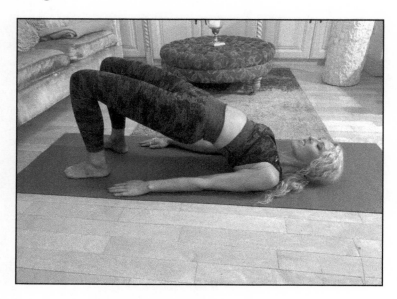

Aim – to improve the mobility of the lumbar spine, to strengthen the hamstrings and the buttocks. **Repetitions-10**

Lie face up

Bend your knees, keeping your feet flat on the floor

Keep your arms by your sides, palms down

Breathe in

Pull your shoulder blades down towards your ribs

Elongate your spine

Contract your abdominal muscles

Breathe out

Lift your pelvis about 15 cm off the floor

Press your feet down into the floor

Repeat 10 times

The 'V'

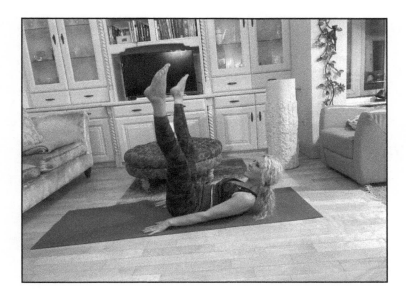

Aim – to strengthen the **abdominals** and quadriceps.

Repetitions – 10

Lie on your back in a good posture, feet a hip's width apart, arms out to the side, palm down at shoulder height

Tighten your abdomen

Breathe out

Bring your legs up to a vertical position, knees directly above your hips, and feet crossed at the ankles

Breathe in

Opening your legs into a wide V and breathe out to bring your legs back to the centre

Repeat 10 times

One Hundred Advanced

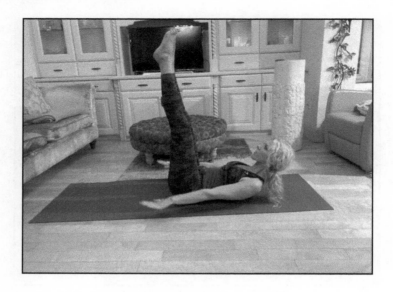

Aim – to strengthen the abdomen and work the thighs.

Count of 100

Lie on your back, arms by your sides, toes lightly pointed

Breathe out

Curl your head and shoulders off the floor,

Raise your arms off the floor and parallel with it

Breathe in

Tighten your abdomen

Lift your legs 15 cm off the floor

Keep legs straight, with your inner thighs together and your toes pointed

Breathe in for 5 seconds, beat your arms up and down over a range of 15 cm, 100 times.

Pelvic Tilt

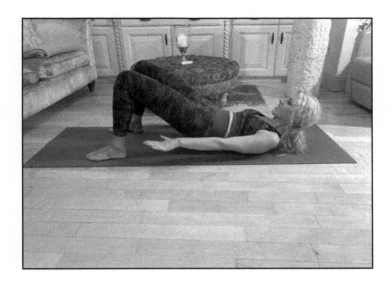

Aim – to improve spine mobility and stability

Repetitions-10

Lie on your back, legs a hip's width apart and bent

Lengthen your spine and tighten your abdomen

Breathe out

Lift your pelvis off the ground and press into your feet

Breathe in

Return to start

Repeat 10 times

Pilates Push Up

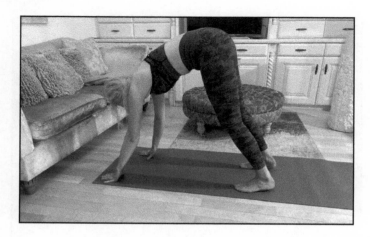

Aim – to improve strength in arms, chest and upper back and flex the hamstrings

Repetitions -5

Stand with your feet a hip width apart

Tighten your abdomen

Breathe out

Bending forward to place your palms on the floor

Keep your legs straight

Breathe in

Walk your hands forward to create a bridge

Move your body forward into a standard press up position, hands directly under your shoulders Breathe out

Bend your arms, lowering your hips in line with your body, parallel to the floor

Breathe in as you straighten your arms again

Repeat 5 times

Breathe in as you walk your hands back to your feet and breathe out to return to the start position

Piriformis Stretch

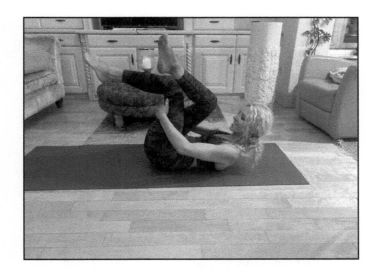

Aim – to release the lumbar spine

Lie on your back, checking for a neutral spine

Keep your legs a hip width apart and bend your knees,

Keep your feet flat on the floor

Cross your right leg over your left thigh

Keep your right hip loose

Bring your left leg up so that your left knee is over your left hip

Hold your left thigh with both hands linked

Draw your left leg towards your chest, using your upper back muscles

Hold this position for 20 complete breaths

Return to start position

Repeat on opposite side

Plié

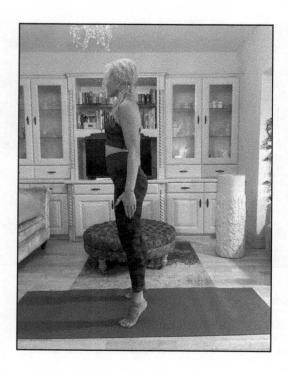

Aim – to tone the legs

Repetitions – 10

Stand in a good posture, feet a hip's width apart

Lengthen your spine

Using your thigh muscles

Turn your feet into a V shape

Keep your spine straight

Breathe in

Breathe out, bending your knees, keeping your heels on the floor

Breathe in, standing tall and then rising onto your toes

Breathe out and return your heels to the floor

Repeat slowly, 10 times.

Psoas Stretch

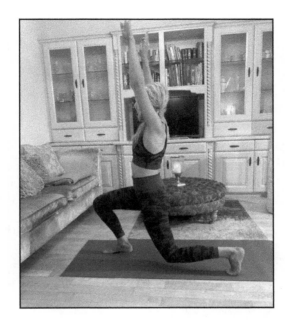

Aim- to increase flexibility in the hips

Repetitions 1+1

Stand in a good posture, spine neutral

Keep your feet a hip's width apart

Face forward

Tighten your abdomen

Take a long step forward with your right leg

Keep your right knee above your right ankle

Extend your arms upwards

Lower your left knee to the floor

Hold this position for 20????

Complete breaths

Return to the start position

Change legs and repeat

Quadriceps Stretch

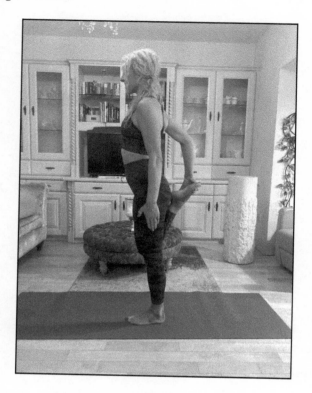

Aim – to stretch the quadriceps muscles

Repetition 1 +1

Stand in a good posture, spine neutral

Keep your feet a hip's width apart, face forward

Tighten your abdomen

Bend your right knee, taking your foot up behind you

Hold your ankle with your right hand

Keep both knees aligned and your spine straight

Hold this position for 60 seconds

Repeat on the other leg

Hamstring Stretch

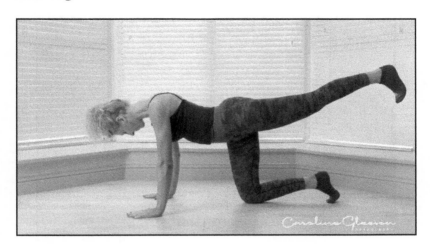

Aim – to lengthen the back of the thigh

Repetition – 5 +5

Stand upright in a good posture, hands linked lightly behind your back

Step forward on one leg

Keep the front leg straight, heel on the ground

Keep your weight on your back leg and bend the knee of the back leg

Lean forward from the hip until you feel the stretch in the back of your front thigh

Hold this position for 10 seconds, change legs

Repeat 5 times on each leg

Triceps Lift

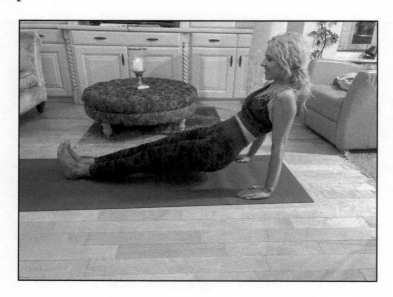

Aim – to strengthen the triceps muscles in the back of the arms

Repetitions- 10

Sit in a good posture, with your legs together and straight in front of you

Put your hands just behind you, palm down so that you can lean back onto them, elbows bent Tighten your abdomen

Breathe out

Push up with both arms, and lift yourself off the floor

Breathe in and lower yourself back to the floor

Repeat 10 times

Oblique Curl up

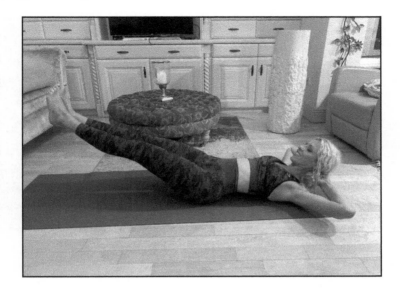

Aim- to strengthen the abdominal muscles

Repetitions – 5+5

Lie on your back and fold your arms behind your head, clasping your hands and leaving your elbows open

Breathe in

Bring your knees up, feet flat on the floor and a hips width apart

Tense your abdomen

Breathe out

At the same time, take your legs up to a 45-degree angle, keeping them straight

Breathe in

Draw up your right shoulders towards your left knee, bending your left knee to meet it

Breathe out

Change sides

Repeat 5 times on each side

Criss – Cross

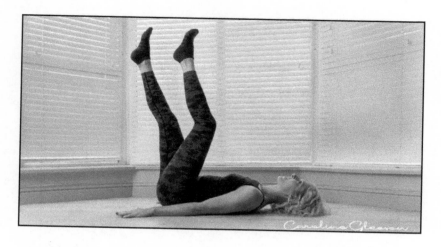

Aim- to rotate the spine and work the abdominal muscles.

Repetitions- 10 + 10

Lie on your back

Lift your left leg about 15 cm off the floor

Bend your right leg up towards your chest so that your knee is above your hip

Put your hands behind your head with your elbows open

Breathe out

Twist your torso to bring your left elbow towards your right knee

Breathe in

Change legs whilst twisting your torso to bring your right elbow towards your left knee

Do not pull on your head

Repeat 10 times with each leg

Double Leg Kicks

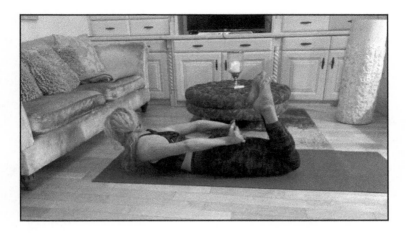

Aim- to open the shoulders and chest, strengthen the spine and tone the buttocks and thighs **Repetitions – 8**

Lie on your front

Turn your head to one side

Link your hands loosely behind your back

Breathe in

As you kick your feet up towards your buttocks

Hold for 3 seconds

Breathe out

As you lower your legs nearly to the floor

Extend your arms towards your feet, keeping your hands clasped

Arch your upper body away from the floor

Breathe in

Return to start

Repeat 8 times

Shoulder Bridge

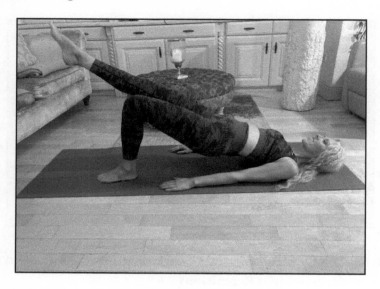

Aim- to strengthen the lumbar spine, gluteals and hamstrings.

Repetitions- 5 + 5

Lie on your back, feet a hip's width apart

Bend your knees, keeping your feet flat on the floor

Breathe in

Tighten your abdomen

Breathe out

Lift your pelvis so that you have a straight line from chest to knees

Breathe in, extending your right leg to a vertical position

Breathe out, lowering your right leg until your knees are level

Breathe in

Return to start position

Change sides

Repeat 5 times on each leg

Chapter 5

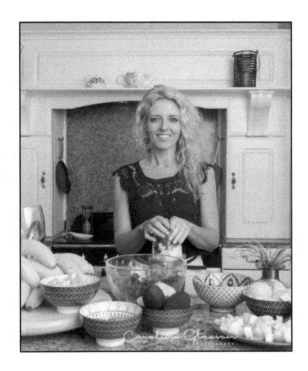

Health Benefits to Delicious Homemade Recipes

The delicious taste from smoothies not to mention the extraordinary health benefits makes it an awesome treat for one's mind, spirit and body. Smoothies just cheer up the senses and give one a good start to the day, paving the way to good health, beautiful skin and a healthy mind.

Lose Weight with a Daily Smoothie

A Smoothie can help one lose excess body weight and help prevent the sugar cravings. The fruits and berries are full of enzymes which help to dissolve body fat and boost the lymphatic system, eliminating toxins from the system and reducing inflammation within the body. Prevents dehydration, water is the most abundant compound both on earth and in the human body.

70 per cent of the body is water. A smoothie drink daily is great to replenish the loss of water in one's body.

Keeping the Body Hydrated

Makes You Feel Satisfied

People who try to lose weight often skip the morning meal and end up snacking on food in larger amounts between meals as their sugar levels drop. One can become extremely weak lacking energy and concentration. This can be avoided by having a smoothie made of excellent fruits and flavours. One will stay full for a longer time, feeling full of vitality and will have balanced sugar levels.

Controls Cravings

Smoothies are full of vitamins, nutrients and minerals providing a power booster pack of goodness for the day. A daily smoothie with protein will provide one with nutrients and goodness to prevent the blood sugar level dropping and prevents cravings.

Aid Digestion and Eliminate Toxins

Green leafy vegetables and berries full of essential minerals and vitamins will provide sufficient fibre which will help detox the system and create a smooth elimination of toxins and fluids internally, helping the digestive system to stay healthy.

The Benefits of Antioxidants

Green and white tea is a popular source of antioxidants and can be added to your smoothies.

One can add maca powder with properties to aid skin rejuvenation and help balance hormones to make smoothies rich in antioxidants. These will help prevent a lot of diseases and ill health.

Boost Immunity

It refers to the ability of the body to fight against pathogens and diseases. This natural potential becomes degenerated due to several reasons such as stress, poor nutrition, lack of sleep, excess caffeine and alcohol.

Smoothies made of ingredients that include nutrients like beta-carotene, vitamins and minerals help boost the immune system and enhance one's overall health.

Sleep Disorders

A healthy breakfast accompanied by a smoothie made of bananas, avocado, kiwi, oats, almond and oat. Milk provides calcium and magnesium in large amounts. This induces sleep and helps maintain healthy sleeping patterns.

Skin-Health

As one may know, food containing carotenoids, like mango, watermelon, pineapple and pumpkin, are highly beneficial for the overall skin health and complexion. Therefore, smoothies that contain these ingredients help the skin to glow.

Provides Liquid Food Benefits

Health and nutrition experts worldwide suggest consuming liquid food for better digestion. Smoothies contain blended fruits and vegetables.

In liquid form they make it easier for the body to break them down, soothing your digestive tract.

Detoxifies the Body

Foods like

- Cabbage
- Kale
- Spinach
- Broccoli
- Brussels sprouts
- Garlic
- Papaya
- Beetroot
- Celery
- Blueberries
- Grapefruit

All help cleanse one's blood, get rid of several toxins accumulated in the body tissues.

Boosts Brain Power

It is quite evident that certain fruits and vegetables increase brain power, boost memory function, mental alertness and concentration which are greatly enhanced by ingredients like

- Coconut
- Hemp seeds
- Avocado
- Quinoa

They are all rich in omega-3 fatty acids which will lower blood pressure and reduce inflammation.

Smoothies with these ingredients help the brain to work effectively.

Controls Mood Swings

An abundance of fruits and vegetables serve an excellent stress booster from the taste to the colour of these delicious smoothies made from fresh ingredients. In return they will relieve stress and give one that feeling of health and vitality.

Fights Depression

Fresh vegetables and fruits are rich in

folic acid like

- broccoli
- spinach
- kale
- bananas

They are all full of goodness and help to balance hormones, blood sugar levels and improve one's over-all health.

Calcium

A regular intake of calcium in the right amount is essential for bone and tooth health. Moreover, it can affect hair growth, nail growth and

Have a Healthy Heart.

Smoothies prepared with dairy or fortified dairy alternatives serve as a great source of calcium for the body.

Smoothie for Health

A daily smoothie will help to boost one's immunity, fuel the body and mind with essential vitamins and minerals.

- Keep blood sugar in check
- Prevents heart disorders
- Prevents dehydration
- Helps with weight management
- A source of fibre
- A source of calcium
- Improves bone health
- High source of antioxidants
- Enhances immunity
- Improves skin
- Detoxifies the body
- Boosts brain power

Frozen Berries Smoothie

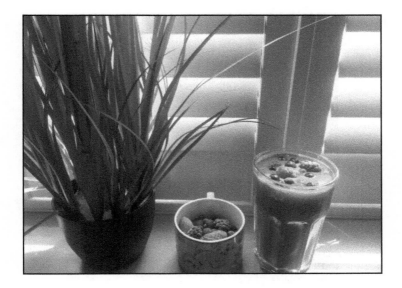

Ingredients:

450g bag frozen berry
450g pot fat free vanilla yogurt
100ml almond milk
25g pre-soaked porridge oats
2 teaspoons of honey

Method:

Whisk berries, yogurt, milk together to a smooth mixture, stir in the pre-soaked porridge oats.

Health Benefits:

- Loaded with vitamins and minerals
- Fights inflammation
- High in fibre
- Loaded with antioxidants

Pineapple Smoothie

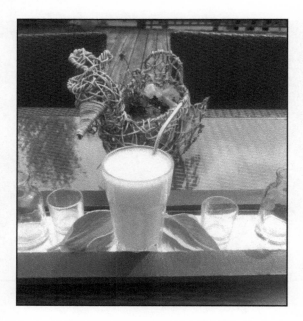

Ingredients:
1 pineapple
1 Banana
450g orange juice
450g Greek natural yogurt

Method:

Whisk all the ingredients together

Health Benefits:

- Contains enzymes that ease digestion
- Boosts one's immunity
- Suppresses inflammation
- Ease symptoms of arthritis
- Contains antioxidants
- Loaded with nutrients and minerals

Avocado Smoothie

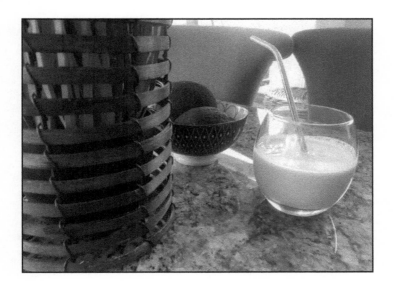

Ingredients:

1 Avocado
4 teaspoons of Vanilla yogurt
1 teaspoon of Honey
2 teaspoons of Protein powder
½ cup of Milk

Method:

Whisk all ingredients until smooth

Health Benefits:

- Avocados are loaded with heart healthy monounsaturated fatty acids
- Loaded with fibre and low in carbohydrates
- Can lower cholesterol
- Reduces blood triglycerides (contains fatty acids)
- Powerful antioxidants and helps prevent cancer cells

Mango Smoothie

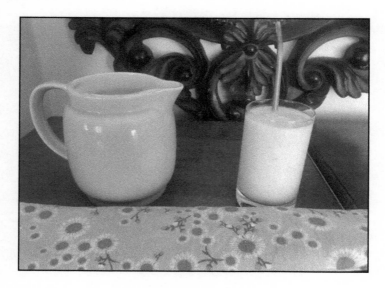

Ingredients:

1 Mango
1 Banana
500ml Orange Juice
4 ice cubes

Method

Whisk all ingredients until smooth

Health Benefits:

- Aids healthy clear skin
- Promotes a healthy gut
- Lowers cholesterol
- Aids weight loss
- Helps aid digestion
- Boosts immunity

Need to detox!

Make one beetroot smoothie daily for one week

Beetroot Smoothie

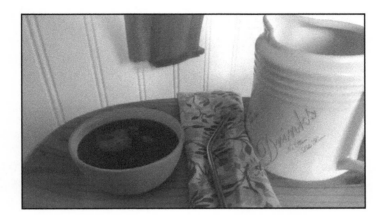

Ingredients:

1 Apple
1 Beetroot peeled and grated
1 Carrot
4 Leafy spinach
½ glass of water

Method:

Whisk all ingredients until smooth

Health benefits:

- Improves energy
- Loaded with nutrients
- High in fibre, potassium and iron
- Improves blood flow
- High in vitamin C

It lowers Blood Sugar and is very healing for the gut.

Cinnamon Smoothie

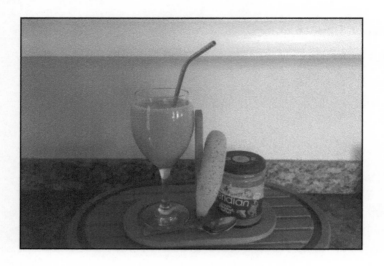

Ingredients:

1 Banana
3 teaspoons of Natural Greek Yogurt
½ Glass of Milk
1 teaspoon of Peanut Butter
1 teaspoon of Cinnamon

Method:

Whisk all ingredients until smooth

Health benefits:

- A Powerful anti-diabetic effect
- Anti-inflammatory
- Lowers blood sugar
- Reduces the risk of heart disease
- Builds and strengthens the immune system

Cherry Mango Smoothie

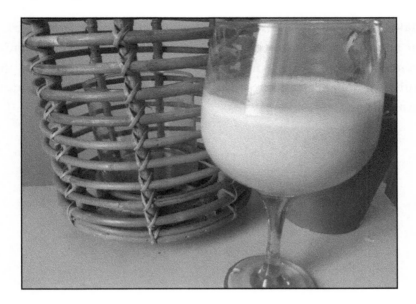

Ingredients:

250g Frozen mango chunks
450g Frozen cherries
½ glass of milk
½ glass of orange juice

Method:

Whisk all ingredients until smooth.

Health Benefits:

- Strengthens the immune system
- Loaded with vitamin A and C
- Antioxidants, helping to prevent cancer
- Anti-inflammatory properties

A TIP

Make it easier and more cost effective. Purchase frozen fruit for smoothies. It is more convenient to take some frozen fruits from the fridge at any time of the day. It is also healthy and the fruits when harvested are preserved, locking in all their vitamins, minerals and antioxidants.

About the Author

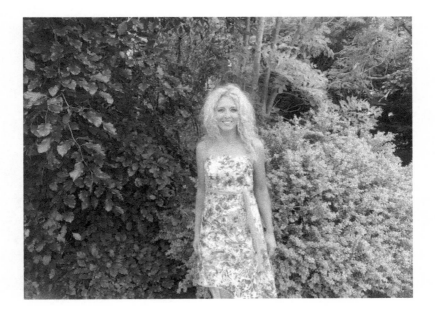

I teach for LCETB (Limerick Clare Educational Training Board).

My journey began after completing my degree in business. I wanted to help people in whatever way possible. I continued studying beauty and body therapy, physical therapy along with a number of holistic therapies such as reflexology, pilates, yoga, medical acupuncture in both western and eastern medicine and ayurvedic medicine. I am working in the health and beauty industry for over twenty-three years offering a range of treatments to ensure my clients and patients health conditions and concerns are fully adhered to.

As a tutor, I enjoy sharing my knowledge and experience within the classroom and encouraging many learners to self-grow through the world of health and wellness. My aim is to immerse each student into this area of healing and fulfilment from the very beginning, sowing the seed of well-being and self-care to ensure one to become a balanced, caring individual, able to share a wealth of knowledge, beliefs and stories in their field of work.

Lightning Source UK Ltd.
Milton Keynes UK
UKHW012333130821
388823UK00001B/301